# Teaching Palliative Care

## A practical guide

Edited by

David Jeffrey

Radcliffe Medical Press

**Radcliffe Medical Press Ltd**
18 Marcham Road
Abingdon
Oxon OX14 1AA
United Kingdom

**www.radcliffe-oxford.com**
The Radcliffe Medical Press electronic catalogue and online ordering
facility.
Direct sales to anywhere in the world.

---

British Library Cataloguing in Publication Data

A catalogue record for this book is available from the British Library.

ISBN 1 85775 579 0

Typeset by Joshua Associates Ltd, Oxford
Printed and bound by TJ International Ltd, Padstow, Cornwall

# Teaching
# Palliative
# Care

**A** practical guide

# Contents

List of contributors                              viii

Acknowledgements                                    ix

Introduction                                         1

1 The teaching approach                              5

   Principles of adult learning       6

   What makes a 'good' teacher?       8

   The PEGG philosophy                9

2 Planning and organising                           11

   Planning a study day              13

   Important planning decisions      15

   Audio-visual equipment            17

   Last minute fine-tuning           20

   Evaluation and closing            20

3 Teaching techniques: Introductions                21

   Groundrules                       22

   Icebreakers                       23

   Physical activities               24

   Creative activities               25

   Illustration                      26

   Practical exercises               27

**4 Teaching techniques: Presentations**                    29

Critiquing a paper                                          30

The lecture                                                 32

Debates                                                     35

**5 Teaching techniques: One-to-one and small group        37
work**

Tutoring                                                    38

Clinical bedside teaching                                   39

Mentoring and supervision                                   42

Facilitating skills in small group work                     44

**6 Teaching techniques: The communication skills          49
ladder**

The communication skills ladder                            50

Interactive video                                          50

Goldfish bowl                                               53

**7 Teaching techniques: Role playing and sculpting**      59

Role play                                                   60

Variants of role play                                      61

Sculpting                                                   62

**8 Evaluation**                                           69

Why is the evaluation required?                            70

Who should do the evaluation?                              70

What aspects of the programme should be evaluated?         71

What kind of measurement will be used?                     72

When will it be done?                                      72

What to do with the evaluation                            72

9 Training the trainers                                    75

Training the trainers: Day 1                              76

Training the trainers: Day 2                              80

10 Lesson plans                                            83

Lesson plan: What is palliative care?                     84

Lesson plan: Pain control                                 87

Lesson plan: Breaking bad news                            90

11 Conclusions                                             93

References                                                 97

Index                                                      99

# List of contributors

## Editor

**Dr David Jeffrey** MA FRCP(Edin)
*Macmillan Lead Consultant in Palliative Medicine*
Three Counties Cancer Centre, Cheltenham General Hospital, Cheltenham

*Honorary Senior Lecturer*
Department of Palliative Medicine, University of Bristol, Bristol

## Contributors

**Denise Barr** BSc(Hons)
*Clinical Nurse Specialist, Hospital Palliative Care Support Team*
Three Counties Cancer Centre, Gloucestershire Royal Hospital, Gloucester

**Mark G Brennan** BA MA AKC DHMSA FCollP FRSH
*Lecturer in Medical and Dental Education*
University of Wales College of Medicine, Cardiff

**Dr Radi Counsell** MD MRCP FRCR
*Consultant Clinical Oncologist*
Three Counties Cancer Centre, Cheltenham General Hospital, Cheltenham

**Sandra Flanagan**
*Administrator, Palliative Care Team*
Three Counties Cancer Centre, Cheltenham General Hospital, Cheltenham

**Kathy Keogh** BA(Hons) Dip Pall Care
*Clinical Nurse Specialist, Palliative Care Hospital Support Team*
Three Counties Cancer Centre, Cheltenham General Hospital, Cheltenham

**Ray Owen** BA(Hons) MSc CPsychol
*Clinical Psychologist in Palliative Care and Macmillan Lead Clinician for Psychosocial Services in Cancer*
Three Counties Cancer Centre, Gloucestershire Royal Hospital, Gloucester

# Acknowledgements

Thanks to the enthusiastic members of the Palliative Care Education Group Gloucestershire (PEGG) who give so generously of their time, to the BUPA Foundation for the Communication Award 1998, and to all who have contributed their wisdom to this book.

# Introduction

Multidisciplinary palliative care has been defined as:

> *the active total care of patients whose disease is not responsive to curative treatment. Control of pain, of other symptoms, of psychological, social and spiritual problems, is paramount. The goal of palliative care is achievement of the best quality of life for patients and their families. Many aspects of palliative care are also applicable earlier in the course of the illness in connection with anticancer treatment.*[1]

The diverse needs of patients and their families demand a multiprofessional response from palliative care teams. Such a team approach is widely accepted as the optimal model of delivery of palliative care services.[2] However, it is interesting to note that professional education tends to be concentrated within single disciplines. We suggest that a practical approach to teaching and training in palliative care should adopt a multiprofessional team approach in education and training.

Healthcare professionals working in palliative care may feel inhibited from teaching for a number of reasons:

- lack of confidence in teaching skills
- pressures of clinical work
- professional isolation
- lack of teaching experience
- bad teaching experience.

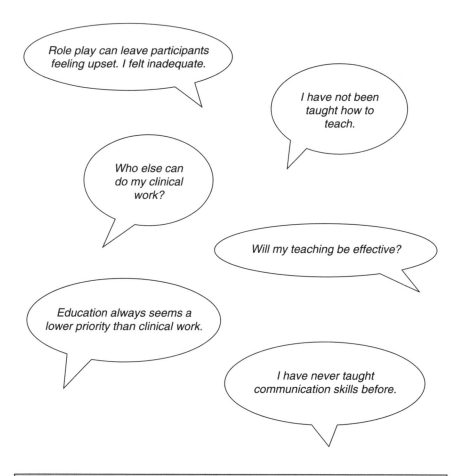

> Role play can leave participants feeling upset. I felt inadequate.

> I have not been taught how to teach.

> Who else can do my clinical work?

> Will my teaching be effective?

> Education always seems a lower priority than clinical work.

> I have never taught communication skills before.

**The aims of this guide are:**

- To encourage busy clinicians to teach by increasing their confidence in their training abilities.
- To provide a practical resource of teaching techniques.

This practical guide has developed from the collective experience of the Palliative Care Education Group for Gloucestershire (PEGG).[3] This is a multidisciplinary group of doctors, nurses, social workers, psychologists, members of other professions allied to medicine and members of the clergy. The contributors to this book reflect the multidisciplinary composition of PEGG.

Teaching and learning together should be fun and this guide emphasises the importance of establishing a relaxed learning environment. People do not learn or retain information when they are apprehensive or frightened.

Teaching and learning should take place in an environment where everyone's view is respected, where the positive is emphasised before the negative and where people feel safe to disclose areas of difficulty – a culture of positive critique.

Using such an approach facilitates the development of healthcare professionals who are both competent and compassionate and who are inspired to continue to develop their own education.

The guide describes our approach to team teaching, planning, teaching methods and evaluation. In each chapter, we present a menu of techniques which have been tried and tested by the PEGG group. Each subject chapter closes with an example of a lesson plan. This guide is not a blueprint of 'the right way to teach' but a toolbox of techniques from which clinical teachers may select ideas and adapt them to their own teaching style.

We hope this guide will be of practical help to healthcare professionals teaching palliative care, whether in hospitals, hospices or in the community.

# Chapter 1

# The teaching approach

Education should be liberating and broadening. It should affect our daily lives and the way we practice our profession. Many doctors and nurses feel guilty if they read journals or textbooks during working hours, as if this type of learning should only be done at home as a leisure activity rather than treated as an integral part of their clinical practice. Learning as an adult is very different from being at school. A better understanding of the principles of adult education can enable all healthcare professionals to become lifelong learners, capable of enjoying teaching and learning.

There have been changes in both medical and nurse education, which have involved moves away from the traditional model of teaching passive learners. Historically, the assimilation of factual information was emphasised and interaction between teacher and learner was minimal. Consider a lecturer talking to a large audience of medical students in a lecture theatre. The teacher presents the student with a quantity of facts. The student records these facts as 'notes', learns the notes, and regurgitates them in exams. Nowadays, learning should be an active process, which broadens the learner's horizons and enables the learner to take responsibility for his or her own professional development.

# Principles of adult learning

At the centre of theories of adult learning lie four basic assumptions:[4,5]

1  Adults both desire and enact a tendency towards self-direction – we all enjoy being involved in decisions which affect our future.

2  Adults' experiences are a rich resource for learning. Adults therefore will learn more effectively through experiential methods of learning, such as small group work and problem solving. Adults need to see why teaching material is relevant to their work.

3  Adults are aware of specific learning needs generated by real life tasks or problems. They need to be encouraged to discuss needs. Saying, 'I don't know' is the first step to gaining new knowledge.

4  Adults are competency-based learners: they wish to apply their newly acquired skills or knowledge to their immediate circumstances. Learning new skills is often uncomfortable, but if the environment is safe, learners can practice new skills

without embarrassment. We need to create an environment where 'it is OK not to feel OK'.

To satisfy these key requirements, we must discard passive learning and develop a new approach.

Knowles has identified seven principles of adult learning which facilitate the shift of responsibility for change to the learner, and which need to be addressed by organisers of adult learning programmes.[6]

1 Establish a physical and psychological climate or ethos of learning.
2 Involve learners in mutual planning and curriculum directions.
3 Involve learners in diagnosing their own needs.
4 Involve learners in formulating their own learning objectives.
5 Involve learners in identifying resources and devising strategies using these resources to accomplish their objectives.
6 Help learners carry out their learning plans.
7 Help learners apply qualitative evaluation methods to their learning.

A study of educational needs of general practitioners and community nurses concluded that 90% of GPs and 95% of community nurses thought that multidisciplinary teaching sessions would be helpful.[7] Barclay *et al.* concluded from their study that 'there is a continuing need for medical education in palliative care'.[8] On the other hand, Macleod and Nash found that the majority of general practitioners were uncomfortable with experiential methods and preferred didactic teaching.[9] Specialist palliative care requires effective multidisciplinary and interdisciplinary teamwork. It is therefore surprising that, generally, medical and nursing education programmes pursue rigidly separate pathways.

Good learners are:

- selective but also experimental
- prepared to change the way they learn
- inquisitive and open to new ideas
- prepared to share knowledge with others
- motivated and enthusiastic
- organised and committed
- broad minded
- able to accept both praise and constructive suggestions for improvement.

## What makes a 'good' teacher?

It is helpful to ask a small group exploring adult education methods to think back to their best ever experience of education and to identify what made that experience special. Most people can remember a particular inspirational teacher who stimulated their interest in a subject, whom they perhaps saw as a role model or mentor. From our experience, learners typically identify the following qualities:

- enthusiasm
- friendliness
- an interest in students and learners
- competence
- knowledge
- confidence
- charisma
- willingness to prepare well
- patience
- ability to listen.

Perhaps the most important quality is the ability to make the learner feel valued. We are all colleagues together and we are all learning from each other. This positive learning environment and sense of community is crucial in the multidisciplinary approach to teaching.

# The PEGG philosophy

Drawing on the experiences of teachers and learners, the PEGG team have developed a philosophy which aims to create the best possible learning environment.

An integral part of PEGG philosophy is positive critique. This recognises that praise and constructive criticism are much more effective than humiliation in education and professional development.

We acknowledge that we learn a great deal during our clinical work from both colleagues and patients. The PEGG approach recognises that we all learn from each other – teachers from different disciplines and learners.

Teachers are facilitators, not just transmitters of facts. Teaching is an active problem-solving process, firmly rooted in clinical practice, enabling learners to quickly grasp the relevance of the material to their work.

The aim of the teaching is to produce practitioners who are both scientifically competent and sensitive to the (often unspoken) needs of patients and their families. Teachers thus need to be role models and show that they are flexible, sensitive and committed to a team approach.

Such team working involves adaptability. It is not hierarchical, pious or grim. Leadership is necessary to give direction, but teachers and learners set their objectives together.

Interactive methods engage learners in their own education, and motivate them to critically evaluate their own beliefs and expectations. Healthcare professionals need to have the confidence to share difficulties with colleagues. In this way they can enhance their professional judgement and make professional decisions in complex and uncertain clinical situations.

The teaching techniques described in this book can help both the teacher and the learner to engage in this active learning process.

# Chapter 2

# Planning and organising

The success of a clinical intervention will often depend upon the time and care taken in the initial assessment. In the same way, the success of a teaching session depends on the time and care taken in the initial planning. Excessive planning and rehearsal can increase the time commitment involved in teaching, to the point of acting as a deterrent for busy clinicians. However, efficient planning is essential for good quality education, bringing benefits to both teacher and learner.

Effective planning increases the teacher's confidence that:

- the aims and objectives of the session are clear
- a competent and enthusiastic teaching style will be presented
- the content will be comprehensive, co-ordinated and not repetitive
- time management has been addressed
- any potential problems arising within small groups have been anticipated
- the skills of members of the teaching team have been pooled and shared
- the risk of mixed messages from different teachers will be minimised
- support will be available from fellow teachers
- constructive feedback from colleagues will be available at the end of the session
- teachers can 'cover' each other
- teachers can learn from each other
- time can be saved in future by using (and if necessary amending) the teaching plan.

Planning needs to occur in both team and individual settings. Important factors may include ensuring that everybody involved in the teaching meets together to agree content and format, that practical issues are addressed, and that any activities such as role play are rehearsed.

As in any team activity, it is important that a key person (leader) is clearly identified for each teaching event.

Adequate time needs to be set aside for planning. As a rough guide, we spend about the same time on planning as teaching if the subject is familiar, but about four times as much time is spent on planning a 'new' teaching session as is spent during the session itself.

If a teaching session is well planned, learners will have:

- confidence about participating in the session
- an appreciation that the session will be relevant, and not repetitive or chaotic
- an overview of the structure of the session, enhancing understanding and retention
- a clear understanding of the aims and learning outcomes
- a sense of ownership of the agenda, and commitment to the teaching session
- interest and concentration stimulated with a variety of teaching techniques
- an expectation of being able to gain a variety of perspectives on a clinical problem
- confidence that essential components will not be overlooked
- confidence in the teacher's competence
- involvement in improving future teaching sessions, by providing feedback
- a sense that learning is stimulating and fun.

# Planning a study day

Priorities when arranging a study day include:

- defining the learning need
- appointing the lead facilitator for the day
- appointing the person who will organise the administration of the event.

Arrange a planning meeting between the lead facilitator, the organiser and all the teachers involved in the event.

## PLANNING MEETING AGENDA

✓ Identify learning needs and ideal outcomes.

✓ Date, duration, venue.

✓ Content and allocation of topics to teachers.
This stage may identify a specific need for another teacher with the relevant skills and knowledge to be approached.

✓ Structure of the day.

✓ Choice of teaching techniques.

✓ Audio-visual equipment.

✓ Method of evaluation.

✓ Catering requirements.

✓ Funding.

✓ Sponsorship.

✓ Advertising the event.

All tasks must be clearly allocated.

## ADMINISTRATIVE CHECKLIST FOR A STUDY DAY

✓ Meet with leader and speakers for the day.

✓ Organise dates.

✓ Book venue.

✓ Advertise the event.

✓ Organise speakers.

✓ Arrange sponsorship if appropriate.

✓ Prepare a teaching timetable.

✓ Schedule lunch and tea breaks with caterers.

✓ Send out application forms.

✓ Confirm applications.

✓ Arrange catering (check special dietary requirements).

✓ Check presentation equipment.

✓ Prepare a programme.

✓ Organise PGEA/CME/Certificates of attendance.

✓ Prepare an attendance list for facilitators.

✓ Prepare registration form for delegates' signature.

✓ Handouts.

✓ Evaluation forms.

# Important planning decisions

## Identifying learners' needs

Plan how to present the aims of the day and the learning outcomes. Negotiate with the learners to check that this meets with their learning needs. Be prepared to be flexible and adapt the plan. Good planning does not mean rigid planning but rather gives the teacher the confidence to be flexible and respond to the learners' agenda.

## Choice of teaching technique

The teachers need to plan which techniques they are going to use. For example, the opening icebreaker needs to fit the subject for the day. If the session is on communication skills, the teacher needs to decide whether a teaching video or role play would be more appropriate. Time needs to be allocated for discussion and reflection. It is better to cover a few subjects thoroughly than to rush through a busy agenda which leaves students confused. Facilitators need to decide how they are going to help if participants become distressed. They need to plan for flexibility, to be ready to change the agenda if the learners identify different needs.

Commonly used teaching formats include:

- **The lecture** – suitable for teaching factual knowledge or research findings to a larger audience; tends to be less interactive, mainly requires good presentation skills.
- **The workshop** – usually a half or full day covering a theme and involving different teaching techniques, including presentations and opportunities for small group discussion; more interactive.
- **The seminar** – often involves the presentation of a paper, either by the facilitator or by a learner, which is then discussed by the group. This is a more interactive format and tends to involve a smaller group.
- **Small group teaching** – highly interactive teaching involving groups of people (usually between 6 and 12) which is interactive and experiential. Discussion and reflection is stimulated by clinicians using their own clinical experience.
- **The tutorial** – specialised small group work (1–6 people). Tutorials are a useful way of giving feedback, encouraging reflective practice and looking in depth at specific topics.
- **The journal club** – a specialised form of small group work which involves systematically critiquing a piece of research evidence or review and presenting it to other learners.
- **Clinical 'bedside' teaching** – generally one-to-one or very small group work which involves role modelling and teaching of practical clinical skills and communication skills.
- **Supervision** – there can be either one-to-one supervision between a mentor and supervisee or small group supervision where professionals of a similar level and experience working within the same discipline meet with a supervisor on a regular basis. The purpose is to encourage reflective practice. This is probably the most interactive form of teaching.

## The venue

Certain kinds of teaching activities are best delivered in certain kinds of environment. For example, small group role play is difficult to deliver in a tiered lecture theatre, and tables may act as a barrier to small group discussions. If at all possible, it is best to visit a new venue before the teaching event.

---

**VENUE CHECKLIST**

✓ Are the physical surroundings appropriate?

✓ Is it warm enough?

✓ Is there enough light?

✓ Is there privacy to protect the learners' right to confidentiality?

✓ Is it possible for everyone to sit?

✓ Are the seats arranged as you wish?

✓ Will everyone be able to see and hear clearly?

✓ Are there other rooms available for small group work?

✓ Are there likely to be distractions, e.g. from other nearby groups?

✓ Check the procedure in the event of fire.

✓ Check the toilet location.

---

# Audio-visual equipment

So often excellent presentations fail because the teacher is unfamiliar with the presentation technology or the equipment fails. It is better for the teacher to work with audio-visual equipment that he or she is familiar with than to struggle with a complicated and unfamiliar system. For example, it may be more appropriate to use overhead projectors (OHPs) effectively than to use a computer-based presentation system badly. There are courses available to learn how to use different computer-based presentation techniques. If handled well they are clear and impressive. However, if they are too gimmicky, they can be distracting.

It is important to match the presentation method to the teaching technique used.

| Teaching method | Appropriate AV aids |
|---|---|
| SMALL GROUP | *Flip chart – summarise points*<br>*Video – communication skills* |
| LECTURE – SMALL TO MEDIUM | *OHPs – smaller audience*<br>*Slides – larger audience*<br>*Computer projection, e.g.*<br>*Powerpoint Video – to illustrate*<br>*a point or provide humour* |
| CONFERENCE PRESENTATION | *Slides*<br>*Computer projection*<br>*Video (large scale projection)* |

**VISUAL AIDS CHECKLIST**

✓ What is available?
✓ Does it work?
✓ Do the teachers know how to use it?
✓ Is there a technician available if things go wrong?
✓ How do you contact this person quickly?

## Slides: points to remember

⚠ Slides may illustrate all the points in a talk, or just the salient ones. Plan the lecture and then decide which points need slides. Do not plan the lecture around your slides.

⚠ Make sure that your slides are simple, short and snappy.

Avoid lots of statistics, complicated graphs and too much information. A cartoon is worth a hundred words.

⚠ It is useful to have blank slides for times in the talk when you are discussing a point or summarising what has gone before.

⚠ Always load your own slides – never give them to someone else! There are always numerous helpful hands waiting to take your slides when you arrive. Make sure you have a chance to see them loaded and have a practice run through. It is useful to have your own viewing box and a carousel.

⚠ What will you do if the equipment fails? Have you a backup, e.g. OHPs

## Overhead projection: points to remember

OHPs are useful in small group situations. They are more interactive than slides, and they are also cheaper and more flexible. They are an excellent tool when used by a teacher who has practised using them.

⚠ OHPs that are not professionally produced may give a poor impression.

⚠ The slowly revealed or 'striptease' OHP technique can be intensely irritating.

⚠ OHPs and slides should not be used in the same presentation.

⚠ Remember to switch the projector off when not in use.

## Videos and computer projection: points to remember

⚠ Will your materials definitely work with their system?

⚠ Are you familiar with the content of the video?

⚠ Are you using the same software for computer projection?

# Last minute fine-tuning

It is useful to plan time during the day (e.g. coffee and lunch breaks) when the teachers can meet and make modifications to the day in the light of needs identified by the learners and any other matters. We tend to use these breaks as work time for the teachers rather than for socialising with the learners. Although it is also important to allow time to meet and talk with the learners it can be useful if the teachers go somewhere else so that they are not disturbed whilst undertaking this last minute adjustment. These breaks are also an opportunity for teachers to give each other positive feedback on the sessions covered.

Breaks are a valuable learning opportunity for learners too. Much of the change in attitudes in practice is achieved through informal talks with colleagues. Colleagues get a chance to meet each other and develop links for the future.

# Evaluation and closing

The closing for the day should be planned as carefully as the opening.

- Allow time for participants to reflect on the experience.
- Evaluation forms should be relevant and not too complicated.
- Choose a good closing exercise.
- Plan to finish a little earlier than advertised (especially on a Friday afternoon!).

# Chapter 3

# Teaching techniques: Introductions

One of the biggest barriers to effective communication is the natural reticence of participants to contribute, particularly at the outset of a teaching event. An icebreaker is an activity which aims to promote participation from all members of the group and may well allow group members an element of self-disclosure enabling them to get to know each other better.

# Groundrules

Groundrules are an agreed set of conditions, which the group negotiate and abide by. Their purpose is to allow people to feel confident, secure and relaxed, creating an optimal learning environment.

People do not take in, or retain, new information if they are anxious or apprehensive. Groundrules enable the creation of a safe trusting environment which allows learners to reflect on their own beliefs, values and attitudes without feeling threatened.

It is important to set groundrules in any small group or interactive session when people are exploring communication skills, psychosocial or emotional issues or when there is a potential for self-disclosure. Consequently, it may be necessary to set these before any icebreaker, which may involve self-disclosure.

The process of setting groundrules may make people feel that the whole session is going to be very threatening. So explain that the reason for setting them is that even a simple exercise can trigger personal distress and inhibit learning.

## How to do it

⇒ Explain the reasons for groundrules.

⇒ Set the time limit for groundrules – approximately 5 minutes.

⇒ Ask the group to volunteer rules, which would enable them to feel more confident and relaxed within the session.

⇒ Record these on a flip chart.

⇒ Add any further rules that you think may be helpful.

⇒ Check with the group that they agree to the rules and that the list is complete.

⇒ Display the rules on the wall where they are visible throughout the session.

⇒ Explicitly remind the group of the rules when appropriate, e.g. before a role play.

### Some examples of groundrules

- Confidentiality.
- Honesty.
- Respect for others – involves listening to their views.
- Non-threatening – learners should feel the atmosphere is non-judgemental.
- Positive critique underpins the PEGG philosophy.
- Ability to call time out.

The 'time out' clause gives explicit permission for a member of the group to:

- stay within the group but not contribute.
- ask for a change of scenario or clinical example.
- leave the group with the second facilitator checking whether they are OK.

If participants wish to leave the group for a loo break rather than under the time out clause, it is important that they make this explicit so that the second facilitator does not follow them out!

If important groundrules are omitted by the group, e.g. confidentiality, be prepared to add them yourself.

Don't get bogged down – make sure that the groundrules are set within the time limit of 5 minutes.

# Icebreakers

The simplest form of introduction is one in which participants say their name and their place of work, or what their aim is for the day, or one nice thing that has happened to them today, or one non-threatening personal detail ('One thing that makes me unique in this room is . . .'). As a variant of this simple icebreaker, participants may form pairs for a few minutes, get to know their partner and then introduce him/her to the group.

# Physical activities

## Throwing and catching a ball

The group sit in a circle and the game involves throwing a tennis ball to a participant who then says their name. The game continues until everyone in the group has learnt all the group members' names. A variant is the thrower shouting the name of the person he/she is about to throw the ball to.

## Changing seats

This game is useful to split up cliques. The group sit in a circle and the facilitator picks a feature which will divide the group (e.g. everyone wearing brown shoes), and asks them to stand in the centre of the circle. Then the facilitator asks them to return to a different seat from the one they came from. The exercise can be repeated several times using differing criteria for mixing up the group.

## The cards

This game, which can be played during a break, explores the non-verbal ways we react to colleagues whom we consider our seniors or juniors. Each participant has a playing card attached to his or her back. King is highest and 2 lowest; the aces and several of the intermediate cards are removed to highlight differing levels of seniority. Participants then react both verbally and in a non-verbal way to their colleagues according to the status they perceive them to be but without revealing what card they have on their back. Each participant has no idea what their own status is at the outset, but gradually deduces it as, for example, they are offered coffee, or told to go to the back of the queue. The game ends by the facilitator asking the group to line up with the king at one end and the others in descending rank. The players may then look at their cards.

## Hands across the world

This activity is ideal for ending a day on communication skills or teamwork. Participants crowd into the centre of the room facing each other. They reach out to join hands with two others, criss-crossing each others' arms and hands, to form a knot. Next, without letting go of a hand the group must unravel themselves to form a circle. This involves a great deal of bending, kneeling and crawling. It is not suitable for anyone with a limiting physical disability or a back problem.

# Creative activities

## Designing the perfect palliator

This is a useful ending exercise where groups of three to six each have a sheet of flip chart paper and a felt tipped pen. They then draw a mythical palliator who, for example, might have big ears for listening, broad shoulders for taking anger, leaning forward with head tilted looking sympathetic . . . and so on.

## Newspaper articles

Group members are divided into pairs for this introductory ice-breaker. Each pair is given the name of a newspaper or magazine. (We use *Hello, The Financial Times, The Sun, Private Eye, The Guardian* etc.) Participants interview each other for 5 minutes and come up with a headline and short news snippet in the style of the paper which reveals something about their partner. A *News of the World* style report, for example, might be headlined 'Macmillan

Nurse in Bed Row with GP', and continue with a few words to explain this, in the style of the paper.

## True or false

The facilitator announces an unusual fact about him/herself which may be a lie or the truth. The group has to decide whether it's true or false.

## Book, picture, music

Participants may be invited to bring a piece of music with them and play a short piece and then tell the group why it is important for them. This is suitable for small groups of up to 8. Similarly, a favourite book or picture can be discussed.

# Illustration

Since palliative care demands a holistic approach, there is much to be learned from a study of the humanities which is relevant to the care of patients and their families. Poetry, art, videos, literature and dramatic demonstrations give us a glimpse of the world through other people's eyes.

A study of the arts can help people to think more creatively about a problem. It is particularly useful when covering emotional, ethical and communication issues.

There are an infinite number of ways in which you can use illustrations within a teaching session. We have found the following examples helpful.

- Using poetry to discuss issues of attitudes to death and bereavement. For instance, a study of Douglas Dunn's *Elegies*, to gain insights into grief and mourning.
- Using humorous slides, OHPs, or video clips to introduce or conclude a session. For example, if there has been an

emotional session on breaking bad news, it can be helpful to lighten the mood with a short humorous video clip from *Mr Bean, Doctor in the House* or *The Simpsons.*

- Slides of artwork are often useful to stimulate interest and discussion. What is the artist trying to tell us? Why has he/she painted in this way? Does this help us to understand how a patient might feel?

## Points to remember

⚠ Illustrations must be relevant.

⚠ They can have an unexpected emotional charge.

⚠ Beware of causing offence with humorous illustrations.

⚠ Beware of belittling participants with their suggestions.

# Practical exercises

## The eye contact game

This can be used to illustrate the importance of eye contact in communication. Participants go into pairs facing each other. One is asked to be the speaker, the other a listener. The speaker thinks of a subject which really interests her and about which she is prepared to talk for a minute. The listener's task is to listen attentively, without speaking but maintaining good eye contact for the first half minute. At this point the facilitator will give a signal. The listener has then to continue to listen but to progressively decrease eye contact so that when the minute is up the listener is not looking at the speaker at all. The speaker meanwhile has to try to keep talking. Invariably the group breaks into laughter as speakers falter and stop. The group then reflects on how the speaker and listener feel and how often they look away during their professional interviews with patients and families, for example in looking down at notes, computers or writing prescriptions.

## Breaking bad news mannequin

This is an illustration of non-verbal aspects of breaking bad news. A facilitator acts as the bearer of the bad news. The group can place him in any position in relation to the patient, who is another facilitator sitting in a chair. This exercise is a useful way of exploring non-verbal aspects of breaking bad news such as proximity to the patient, facial expression and posture.

## The uncertainty envelope

This is a dramatic illustration of the dilemmas and uncertainties in talking about a poor prognosis, and a way of thinking about issues of prognosis from the patient's perspective. The group members are each given a sealed envelope which looks official and has their name typed on it with a numerical code. For the purpose of the exercise they are asked to suspend their belief in reality and imagine that their envelope contains the date and time of their own death. They are given time to think about this and then asked by the facilitator, 'Do you want to open your envelope?'

Few do want to, and if they do there is only a blank piece of paper inside.

This exercise leads to a useful discussion of the many issues which lie behind the patient's question, 'How long have I got?'

# Chapter 4

# Teaching techniques: Presentations

There are many different forms of presentation. We have chosen three types:

1 *Critiquing a paper*: a useful method of updating a small group on recent research developments or important reviews in palliative care.

2 *The traditional lecture*: sometimes known as 'chalk and talk'.

3 *The formal debate*: a way of exploring the beliefs and values of those involved in palliative care.

# Critiquing a paper

Primary research commonly reports clinical trials, surveys and experiments. Secondary research tends to consist of overviews, guidelines and meta-analysis. Greenhalgh presents a useful hierarchy of evidence of primary studies:[10]

- systematic reviews and meta-analyses
- randomised controlled trials with definitive results (confidence intervals that do not overlap the threshold for clinically significant effect)
- randomised controlled trials with non-definitive results (a point estimate that suggests a clinically significant effect but with confidence intervals overlapping the threshold for this effect)
- cohort studies
- case-control studies
- cross-sectional surveys
- case reports.

Most papers on palliative medicine follow the generally accepted structure of an introduction followed by methods, results and discussion.[10] Papers often have helpful key points, summary points or an abstract which can give you a quick notion of whether the topic is of relevance to your study.

---

**LOOK AT THE METHODOLOGY**

✓ What was the research question?

✓ Is the author's hypothesis clearly stated?

✓ What kind of study is it – is it a quantitative research study or a qualitative study?

✓ Was the design of the study appropriate to the research question?

✓ Does it adequately test the researcher's hypothesis?

✓ Is the sample of a reasonable size?

✓ Are the statistics sound?

✓ Was the study controlled adequately?

In critiquing a paper it is also useful to be familiar with the background work to which the research relates and to be familiar with the authors and the place where they work. It is important to see whether the authors have drawn relevant conclusions from the data and whether there is interesting and useful discussion.

Finally, it is important to make sure that there is no significant conflict of interest noted at the end of the paper. The general style of the paper is also important – is it accessible and easy to read?

## Running a journal club

Journal clubs involve a small group discussion generally lasting about an hour, which is focused on specific scientific papers. A form of journal club which we have found useful is to reflect on clinical problems from the workplace. The problem is identified at one meeting, someone takes responsibility for seeking out the answer to the problem from the evidence base during the next week and brings the articles to the second meeting. Participants take the papers away to read, and these papers are discussed in the third meeting. During each meeting a new problem is introduced, and a new person assigned to find information so that the cycle continues.

JOURNAL CLUB AGENDA

✓ Selecting clinical problem to research (10 minutes).

✓ Presentation of paper to group with photocopy (20 minutes).

✓ Group discussion of last week's paper (30 minutes).

✓ Written conclusion of any change in practice

# The lecture

A lecture is a presentation where participants listen to an account by a speaker and then may or may not have an opportunity to ask questions. Lectures are a useful way of conveying factual knowledge or research findings (rather than skills) and tend to be used for large audiences, e.g. conferences, meetings or undergraduate teaching.

## How to do it

⇒ Plan both content and structure.

⇒ Know the size of your audience, who they are and their level of knowledge.

⇒ Be familiar with and confident about your subject material.

⇒ Be yourself.

⇒ Be enthusiastic about your subject.

⇒ Give a prepared handout at the end of the session.

⇒ Allow plenty of time for questions and discussion at the end.

⇒ Make sure there is a glass of water available.

---

**There is still mileage in the old adage:**

- tell them what you are going to tell them
- tell them
- tell them what you have told them.

---

Become an expert at giving one or two subjects for a presentation and be prepared to say no to requests for topics that you are unfamiliar with. Plan with other speakers so that you do not overlap.

## Points to remember

⚠ You have been invited as a credible expert, don't apologise for yourself.

⚠ Communicate two or three interesting facts.

⚠ Maintain eye contact with your audience.

⚠ It is good to use humour, e.g. cartoons or video clips.

⚠ Clinical anecdotes add interest.

⚠ AV equipment can provide a change of pace.

⚠ Be prepared for AV equipment failure.

## Difficult audiences

Audiences may become bored after about 20 minutes. If this is happening, the presentation can be made more interactive by getting people to discuss a topic in pairs. The presenter can then ask for feedback. It is best not to give handouts at the beginning of the session as people will read while you are speaking and will not pay attention.

| TIPS FOR DEALING WITH DIFFICULT AUDIENCES | |
|---|---|
| *Difficulty* | *Solution* |
| Apathy | Make more interactive |
| Hostile | Acknowledge, involve, maintain eye contact, find out their agenda |
| Restless | Negotiate, make more interactive |
| Small audience | Switch techniques, use small group work |
| Large audience | Adjust techniques |
| Dominant member | Acknowledge, or silence |
| Chatting | Stop and ask why, inform them it is distracting others |
| No questions | May be OK. If you want discussion ask some questions |
| Different knowledge levels | Assess needs carefully and try to meet some |

If the presentation is a lecture which forms part of a conference or study day, it is helpful to have a chairperson to co-ordinate the day.

**CHAIRPERSON'S CHECKLIST**

✓ Be familiar with the programme and timings.

✓ Get in touch with the speakers beforehand.

✓ Have some interesting background information about the speakers.

✓ Introduce the speakers.

✓ Give a time warning before the end of the talk.

✓ Be prepared to initiate questioning.

✓ Acknowledge any hostility in the audience and protect the speaker from this.

The chairperson can ask controversial questions to stimulate debate. He/she also has the authority to shut people up!

## Presentation: an example

*Topic:* **The management of neuropathic pain**

*Audience:* 20 junior doctors

*Venue:* Postgraduate Centre Lecture Theatre

*Time allocated:* One hour

• Self-introduction

• Give summary of the talk

• Show cartoon relating to pain

• Definitions and mechanisms of neuropathic pain using overheads or slides

• Use of clinical case history

• Clear description of the appropriate management of neuropathic pain

- A summary of the session with key points emphasised
- Give handout to take away
- Close with cartoon/slide
- Questions and discussion

# Debates

Debate is a formal structure where an idea, formally phrased as 'the motion' (e.g. 'this house believes that euthanasia should be legalised'), is discussed by two opposing teams in front of an audience. The teams normally consist of two speakers, a proposer and a seconder, and the debate is chaired.

A formal debate requires a great deal of preparation by a group. Two members agree to propose the motion and two agree to oppose it. All members of the group are advised to think about the topic for the debate. A Chair is appointed (often the facilitator).

The debate requires a room with a table, behind which the two teams sit with the Chair between them. The Chair asks the person proposing the motion to speak. He then asks the person opposing the motion to speak. An opportunity for discussion from the audience and then a summing up from the seconders for and against the motion follows. A vote is carried out at the end (for and against, and abstentions). The Chair then announces the result.

Any of these factors can be varied, for instance the debate could be between one person on each side with an audience of participants. In a 'balloon debate', each speaker is given a role and has to justify their continued presence in the basket of a hot air balloon which is sinking.

## When do we use debate?

This is a useful technique for debating ethical issues such as the rationing of limited resources and end of life decisions, such as euthanasia and the feeding and hydration of terminally ill patients. It is a useful way for group members to explore their attitudes, beliefs and values. We have used debates with groups of learners like GP Vocational Training Scheme Registrars, and on residential courses over a weekend.

## Points to remember

⚠ Many people find this technique daunting. It should never be imposed upon a group.

⚠ You need to feel confident that the group is keen to do it.

⚠ This technique is about argument and can be confrontational.

⚠ Ensure you get participation from the floor and make sure everyone contributes.

Chapter 5

# Teaching techniques: One-to-one and small group work

# Tutoring

Tutoring is a specialised form of small group work, which may involve one to six people. The tutor, who has expertise, leads a discussion on a topic, for which the participants have prepared.

Tutoring occurs on a one-to-one basis or in very small groups as a way of giving feedback and encouraging reflective practice. It is a good technique for looking in depth at specific topics and ensuring that the participants have a good grasp of the subject.

Tutoring can be part of an ongoing educational programme or requested as a one off event. Tutorials can allow participants to address their own specific learning needs.

## How to do it

⇒ It is important to use a quiet room with no disturbance from telephone or bleeps.

⇒ The tutor needs to be prepared for the subject.

⇒ The tutor should ask questions, and encourage participants to find an answer for themselves, rather than simply telling them facts (Socratic dialogue).

⇒ Make sure the trainees have adequate time to prepare for the tutorial themselves.

⇒ Keep time boundaries – no longer than 1 hour.

⇒ Set groundrules.

## What to watch out for

⚠ Being unprepared.

⚠ Having participants who have not prepared themselves for the tutorial and are unfamiliar with the subject matter.

⚠ Quiet participants who do not take part.

⚠ People who wish to take over the tutorial.

⚠ People using the tutorial for personal therapy.

## Tutorials: an example

A tutorial for two GP Registrars on the subject of 'Ethical dilemmas of hydration and feeding at the end of life in patients with advanced cancer'.

### Preparation

The GP Registrars are given background references reflecting differing ethical viewpoints. They are directed to read this background material and to think of any dilemmas in this area which they have encountered in their own practice or during their hospital training.

The tutor prepares a case which highlights these dilemmas.

---

**TUTORIAL PLAN**

✓ Remind yourselves of the aims of the session.

✓ Agree a time boundary.

✓ Begin by discussing the background reading and elicit the participants' views.

✓ Identify the areas of interest or difficulty for the learners.

✓ By question and discussion, using case histories as examples and the combined clinical experience, elicit ways of approaching such ethical dilemmas.

✓ Summarise these methods.

✓ Identify implications for future practice.

✓ Identify any future learning needs.

---

# Clinical bedside teaching

Clinical bedside teaching is extremely valuable and best done on a one-to-one basis in palliative care. Bedside teaching involves working with another clinician in a clinical situation, either on the ward, in outpatients, in the GP surgery or in the patient's home, with the patient's consent, and reflecting on the experience afterwards. It is well suited for teaching practical procedures such as clinical examination and communication skills.

## How to do it

Bedside teaching demands an experienced practitioner. The learner needs to be given the background of the situation before meeting the patient. The patient also needs to be prepared to take part in a teaching situation and to give their informed consent.

The teaching may take a variety of forms, either role modelling, where the learner watches the experienced practitioner, or the learner undertaking a practical procedure under the supervision and watchful eye of the experienced teacher. It may involve the learner assessing or examining the patient and then returning to the teacher to talk about their findings later, and reflecting on the consultation.

In some situations, with suitable safeguards of confidentiality and patient consent, bedside teaching can be enhanced by video recording the consultation.

## What to watch out for

 Issues of consent and ethics with the patient.

 Patient confidentiality, particularly if the consultation is being recorded on video.

 Don't exclude the patient when you are talking to the learner. Discussion with the learner alone should be done away from the bedside.

 Take steps to ensure that the learner does not raise issues, in front of the patient, which may be inappropriate to discuss with the patient at that time.

It is critically important to be sensitive to the feelings of the patient throughout any form of bedside teaching and particularly in the area of palliative care.

# Bedside teaching: an example

This example takes place in outpatients. As a Clinical Nurse Specialist you have been asked to support a young 35-year-old woman who has found out at the clinic that she has widespread ovarian cancer, which has now relapsed after her chemotherapy. The Consultant Oncologist has asked you to be involved to support the patient and you are accompanied by a District Nurse on a teaching attachment.

Once the patient and relatives have gone, you point out to the District Nurse the main learning points of the consultation. You then discuss what went well and in what ways it could have been even better, using the system of positive critique.

---

**TEACHING PLAN**

✓ Introduce the patient to the Clinical Nurse Specialist.

✓ Explain the role of the Clinical Nurse Specialist to the patient.

✓ Introduce the District Nurse, and seek the patient's consent for the District Nurse's presence as an observer in the interview.

✓ Ask the patient whether she wishes anyone else to be present.

✓ Find a quiet room.

✓ Use communication skills to listen and explore the patient's fears about the diagnosis and prognosis.

✓ Offer future support, give contact numbers, and offer to liaise with the patient's GP and District Nurse in the community along with the Macmillan Nurse if she/he is involved.

✓ Once the patient and relatives have gone, spend some time with the District Nurse discussing what went well during the consultation and in what ways the consultation could have been even better – a system of positive critique.

✓ Ask the District Nurse whether she has come across similar situations herself and whether there were any particular areas that she found difficult.

✓ Identify future learning needs and how these might be met.

# Mentoring and supervision

Mentoring may be seen as the initiation and development of a learning relationship between teacher and learner designed to help individuals to fulfil their potential and to work effectively through a process of reflective practice. It aims to assist the individual to apply what they have learned and to incorporate their new technical and professional skills effectively in their day-to-day activities. It is a relationship, not just a procedure or activity, where one person professionally assists the career/professional development of another, outside the normal superior/subordinate relationship.

'Clinical supervision' is a term used to describe a formal process of professional support and learning which enables individual practitioners to develop knowledge and competence, assume responsibility for their own practice and enhance consumer protection and the safety of care in complex situations. It is central to the process of learning and to the expansion of the scope of professional practice and should be seen as a means of encouraging self-assessment and analytical and reflective skills.

## The role of the mentor

- To provide support.
- To provide a safe environment.

- To initiate reflective practice.
- To demonstrate own reflective practice.
- To motivate and encourage professional development.
- Joint responsibility.
- To facilitate feedback.

## The responsibilities of the learner

- To willingly and honestly consider their own practice.
- To keep a record/journal of professional development.
- To contribute towards feedback to enhance learning environment.
- Joint responsibility in using time constructively.

Mentoring and clinical supervision sessions should take place in privacy without interruption from visitors, telephones or bleeps. It is recommended that sessions should be a minimum of 30 minutes and a maximum of 1 hour. Any notes taken at the session are the property of the supervisee and are kept for reference.

## Groundrules

- Confidentiality.
- Clear definition of professional issues raised.
- Two way process/partnership based on trust.
- Information not used in other ways, e.g. appraisal.

## How to do it

⇒ Explain/summarise/describe event(s).

⇒ What did you do?

⇒ What did other people do?

⇒ What did you think/feel?

⇒ Why did you choose this event?

⇒ What do you think/feel now?

⇒ What do you want/need to get from discussing the event?

# Facilitating skills in small group work

Facilitating skills in small group work is highly interactive and experiential and relies on clinicians using their own clinical experience with discussion and reflection. Facilitation skills enable an optimal learning environment where participants are relaxed and able to discuss areas which they find difficult in their own practice. Facilitation skills also enable each participant to contribute to the teaching session. The facilitator allows the participants to learn from each other and to reflect on difficult areas of their clinical experience in a safe environment.

Small group work is particularly useful for teaching skills, reflecting on our attitudes and sharing our experiences. It can also be used for teaching factual information but is well suited for less fact-based topics such as communication skills, spirituality and body image. Any topic could be covered with small group work as the main skill in facilitating is to allow the participants to learn from each other and to achieve a balance of contribution from each of the participants.

In contrast to tutoring, the facilitator need not necessarily be an expert on the particular topic being discussed. Facilitation in pairs is preferable to solo facilitation. The facilitators should decide beforehand who will be the main facilitator within the group – the other facilitator will be watching out for participants' reactions. Double facilitation allows less experienced facilitators, who are learning the technique, to gain confidence and shadow the main facilitator.

Single facilitation is quite possible when topics are not likely to arouse any personal distress for any of the participants. If, however, more emotionally charged topics are being discussed, then we would recommend double facilitation.

Good communication skills such as eye contact, listening and using a variety of different techniques such as memorising the Christian (or first) names of the group if at all possible, are required. Reinforce comments made by particularly quiet members of the group so that you achieve a balanced contribution. Eye contact can be used both positively and negatively to draw in contributions from the group.

## How to do it

⇒ Planning.

⇒ An appropriate environment.

⇒ Self-introduction.

⇒ Groundrules.

⇒ Icebreakers.

⇒ Negotiate the agenda and goals for the session.

## Small group facilitation: an example

*Topic*: **Talking with relatives: What are the difficulties? How can we improve?**

*Participants*: A small group of 10 nurses and junior doctors.

*Venue*: Seminar room adjacent to the ward.

*Time allocated*: Two hours.

- Introductions.
- Icebreaker – tell us one thing that makes you unique in the group.
- Explain aims – to identify areas of difficulty in talking to relatives.
- Brainstorm session – list difficulties on a flip chart:
  - lack of time
  - angry relatives

- lack of knowledge of diagnosis or prognosis
- confidentiality
- telephone
- lack of privacy
- collusion.

• Encourage participants to think of clinical situations in which they have had such problems with relatives and recount to the group how they felt at the time. List feelings on the flip chart:

- anger
- inadequacy
- sadness
- uncertainty
- fear
- anxiety
- embarrassment.

• Select a topic to consider in more detail.

This group decides to look at collusion. Group members reflect on clinical situations of collusion. A discussion ensues on how to prevent collusion and ways of promoting openness once collusion is established.

• The co-facilitator uses the flip chart to draw up a model for promoting openness:

- give time to the relative
- acknowledge their motive for protecting the patient
- ask how this is affecting the relative
- establish the emotional costs of maintaining a pretence
- suggest that the relative may already know
- explain why it may be important for the relative to know
- negotiate permission to explore the patient's level of knowledge
- reassure that you will not force information on anybody.

• Closing remarks and verbal evaluation from each group member.

## What to watch out for

⚠ If goals are not clear, discussion can deteriorate into an unstructured ramble.

⚠ Facilitation is about encouraging people to join in, and this can be fun. Sometimes, using humour can go horribly wrong. Be careful that the correct balance is achieved.

⚠ Use self-disclosure very carefully. The material you are introducing may be particularly meaningful for you, but your audience may not feel exactly the same way about it.

⚠ A person may become upset. The group may wish to support this person if he/she remains in the group or the person might want some time out of the group with one of the facilitators. The group should be offered a change in clinical scenario if a particular incident has triggered personal distress. The person affected may find it helpful to express their distress and talk in the group.

⚠ The facilitator may dominate the session. The co-facilitator can gently become more involved and suggest a group exercise. In the space created the dominant facilitator can be encouraged to take a smaller part. Another opportunity to alter behaviour is the feedback session after the participants have gone.

⚠ A participant may wish to take over the group. This can be dealt with by the creative use of eye contact. Look at other members of the group for answers, avoiding eye contact with the person taking over. If subtle measures fail, direct confrontation with the observation, 'You have contributed a great deal, I would like to hear what some of the other members of the group feel' may have a good effect.

⚠ A participant may fall silent. This can be challenging if the member has been contributing and then becomes silent. It may be useful to talk to the person during the next break to establish whether they have a problem. Remember that some people are quiet by nature and may take longer to contribute.

A person may appear bored. Sometimes, the introduction of a game or short group exercise can inject enthusiasm back into a group. Make sure that the session is not running over time.

 A participant may become angry. Time spent with the participant during a break may help to find out why they are feeling anger. Reference to the agreed groundrules may allow a period of time out.

# Chapter 6

# Teaching techniques: The communication skills ladder

Teaching communication skills can be achieved using a variety of techniques. At the heart of this teaching, learners need to be able to practise their communication skills in situations which are as close to real life as possible. This form of practice should be conducted in a safe learning environment. However, many participants feel inhibited about practising communication skills and to meet this difficulty we suggest the use of the communication skills teaching ladder.

# The communication skills ladder

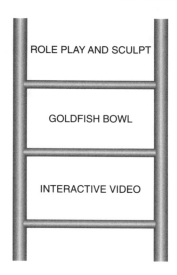

ROLE PLAY AND SCULPT

GOLDFISH BOWL

INTERACTIVE VIDEO

The rationale behind this ladder is that the first steps involve interactive and experiential work but are not at all threatening. As one ascends the steps, the degree of personal participation increases, as does the potential for the learner to feel threatened. However, if we are to improve our communication skills, we need to feel confident enough to practice our skills and to receive constructive feedback from our colleagues.

# Interactive video

This technique involves using a wide variety of teaching videos which feature clinicians, often role playing clinical situations with actors or actresses. Rather than playing the tape straight through, the facilitator encourages active participation by the learners by frequently stopping the tape and asking the learners to suggest possible ways forward in difficult situations before restarting the tape to see what happens.

It is important to note that this technique uses pre-recorded videos, not video consultations or videoing of participants' role plays, which would be discussed in a tutoring situation on a one-to-one basis for feedback.

Interactive videos are best used as a first step in practising communication skills, perhaps with a group who do not know each other very well, or at the beginning of a day on communication skills. They are also very useful for a less experienced group, who do not have their own reservoir of experiences to call upon.

It is important to emphasise the use of positive critique as there is a strong tendency for people to criticise the professionals. It is also worth emphasising in the background remarks how brave the clinicians are to allow their teaching videos to be used in this way and how much more difficult it is to arrive at an appropriate response in the heat of a very realistic role play rather than sitting back and watching it in a small group.

## How to do it

As with all the techniques on the ladder of communication skills, it is best to have two facilitators, one to facilitate the session, the other to watch participants' reactions.

⇒ The facilitator introduces the session and clarifies the aims of the session.

⇒ The groundrules are reviewed.

⇒ The group introduce themselves with a simple technique.

⇒ The facilitator sets the scene of the tape, responds to any anxieties from the learners and checks that the scenario to be discussed is not inappropriate for any of the participants.

⇒ The tape is played and the facilitator pauses the video at frequent points.

⇒ At the end of the video the facilitators check with the participants that they feel comfortable about the scenario.

If the video shows a particularly intense scenario, it is often useful to have a simple ending icebreaker to lighten the atmosphere. In particular, after very sad videos it might be helpful to make a comment about the quality of the acting.

You need to find the right balance of how frequently to stop the tape. Stopping too often can be irritating. Stopping infrequently can mean missing cues for discussion. An added advantage of interrupting the tape frequently is that if it is particularly distressing material this tends to dilute the distress.

---

**FACILITATOR'S CHECKLIST**

✓ Ensure that the videos are available and wound to the correct starting point.

✓ Be familiar with the contents of the tapes.

✓ Be familiar with the machine and the remote control.

✓ Be totally confident that the machine and remote control are functioning.

✓ Use the pause rather than the stop button on the remote control so the tape does not stop or rewind inappropriately.

---

A lot of time can be spent analysing a snippet of the consultation. Participants will often argue that there is not enough time to do this in clinical practice. It is helpful to point to the time indicator and say, 'Well, we are only five minutes into this conversation.'

## Interactive video: an example

---

*Topic*: **Managing collusion**

*Aim*: To promote openness and how to achieve it. Emphasise that as in all palliative care, the relatives require just as much attention and care as the patient.

---

- The facilitator in the small group describes the background of the tape and confirms that it features actors and clinicians role playing.
- The facilitator briefly outlines the scenario and checks with the group whether they find this acceptable and that it does not trigger any personal reactions.
- The facilitator reminds the group of the groundrules and explains that the video will be stopped frequently for discussion.
- The video is set to a clip of a consultant interviewing an elderly lady.
- With frequent stops the group discuss various issues such as eye contact, the angry relative etc.
- Comments are made with the benefit of hindsight.

# Goldfish bowl

The goldfish bowl technique involves the learners sitting in a circle or semi-circle and watching the teaching team carry out a role play. A semi-circle works better than a circle as all participants can see the faces of the characters. A facilitator stops the role play and the learners are asked to suggest words the characters might use to deal with a particular communication problem. They then see their suggestions enacted in the role play and the possible consequences. This technique is best used as a second step in teaching communication skills. It allows participants to give their own ideas on different approaches without feeling threatened or having to take part in a role play themselves.

## How to do it

⇒ Arrange the furniture into a semi-circle or circle with three chairs in the centre, two for the players and one for the facilitator.

⇒ Remind participants of the groundrules.

⇒ State the aims of the session and explain the technique. Participants are allowed to ask any questions or to ask for clarification of the teaching technique.

⇒ The role players (who are familiar with the scenario) practise it up to the first few exchanges until a suitable stopping point is reached. For example, 'How long have I got Doctor?' or 'Am I going to get better?'

⇒ When the facilitator calls a pause, the first people approached to comment on what is going well should be the role players. Then the wider group can comment, and make suggestions as to what they would like to see tried.

⇒ The subsequent role play relies entirely on the contributions of the learners in the bowl. The role players are not giving a demonstration of the 'right way' but acting as a mouthpiece to explore the possible consequences of the learners' suggestions.

⇒ When these suggestions are tried out, the two role players, in role or out of role, can say how they feel about the suggestions and join in the debate.

The goldfish bowl offers a wonderful opportunity to practise different responses using a different language to that which we might ordinarily use in a clinical situation. However, if one of the role players feels that a suggestion is just too alien for their own practice, they, like everyone else in the session, have the right to call time out.

It is useful to script the role play to the point of the trigger question, so that you reach the point fairly rapidly with the group, and exploration of the difficult question can begin. It is quite difficult to manage time here and it is important to stay within the time boundaries.

It is important to have a back-up scenario in case the one you have chosen is in fact inappropriate for one of the group. It is also possible to select the scenario from the group, perhaps earlier in the day, and the teaching team can plan it during a break.

The same groundrules which applied for the interactive video apply here in terms of positive critique. The positive critique is used to identify what was good about a suggestion before identifying things that might have gone better.

## The goldfish bowl: an example

*Topic*: **Exploring difficulties in giving a poor prognosis**

Peter is a 42-year old computer programmer. He is married to Ann and has two young children, Jim and Jill. After six weeks of vague abdominal pains and indigestion, he has been admitted with severe abdominal pain. At laparotomy he has been found to have inoperable pancreatic cancer, which has spread to his liver and throughout the abdominal cavity. His abdomen is closed without any of the cancer being able to be resected other than a small portion of tissue for histology. The histology confirms cancer and the surgeons have told him that no operation is possible. An oncologist has advised him that chemotherapy would be of no benefit. He has now returned home and has made an appointment to see his GP, Dr Black, to discuss what has happened to him in hospital and what happens next.

**TEACHING PLAN**

✓ Review groundrules.

✓ Assign the roles of Peter and Dr Black to team members.

✓ Check that the participants are happy with the scenario.

The two team members have already practised a preamble between Dr Black and Peter to the point where, while Dr Black is looking through the hospital letter, Peter looks up at him and asks, 'How long have I got?'

✓ The role play is allowed to start. When Peter asks his question, the facilitator stops the consultation and says, 'What is actually happening here?'

✓ The team members in role might comment on how they feel the situation is proceeding. What might be going through Dr Black's mind? What might be going through Peter's mind?

✓ The facilitator asks the learners in the circle to imagine that they are Dr Black and to suggest words they like to use or how they would handle this difficult question.

Responses from the learners might include:

'*I would say that it is probably going to be less than a year.*'

'*I don't know, how long is a piece of string?*'

'*That's a very difficult question, Peter, we need to take some time to answer it.*'

✓ A selection of suggestions are acted out.

✓ After practising two or three different suggestions, there is a pause for discussion between Dr Black, Peter and the group members as to what they felt were particularly helpful suggestions.

✓ De-role.

✓ Evaluation.

This technique does run the risk of one participant dominating with suggestions. It is important that the facilitator allows as many participants as possible to put forward suggestions and that there is then group consensus of which suggestions are followed. All suggestions are valued even if not all are implemented. If a suggestion from a participant is met by derision or hostility, it is important for the facilitator to restate the groundrules of mutual respect and that this is an area where more extreme ideas can safely be tried out and explored.

It is particularly important not only to de-role the team players who are role playing but also each member of the group. One technique we suggest is to ask them their name, where they work and one thing they have learned from the teaching session.

Chapter 7

# Teaching techniques: Role play and sculpting

# Role play

Role play involves either participants or facilitators taking on the roles of patients, families and professionals to enact a situation. It can be used to learn communication skills in a safe environment without fear of upsetting patients. Role play is suitable for use in the small group setting with participants who are comfortable with practising communication skills. It can also be used with larger groups who can be split into pairs or trios. Role play takes between 1½ and 2 hours. It is not a technique which is suitable for a short teaching session, even with people who know each other.

## How to do it

Facilitating a small group has been described earlier. Role play can be enhanced with double facilitation, one facilitator leading the group and the other watching out for the reactions of the participants.

⇒ The facilitator explains the situation to be role played and the aims of the session.

⇒ The facilitator checks with the group that this situation is acceptable.

⇒ The facilitator explains the technique of role play and checks participants' previous experience of role play.

⇒ Time boundaries are explained and groundrules are set.

⇒ The facilitator assigns the roles to the participants and starts the role play.

⇒ The role play is stopped frequently by the facilitator, either for discussion of an interesting point or if the facilitator detects that one of the players is having difficulties.

⇒ As soon as the role play is stopped, the facilitator asks the role players, and then the learners, what they feel is going well.

⇒ When the positive things have been discussed, the role players, and then the learners, are asked if there is anything they feel that they could have done better.

⇒ De-role.

Once the role play has been completed, the players must de-role. There are a number of ways to carry out this important part of a role play. We find it useful to have the role players say their own name and say they are not the character name they have been given. Participants change seats and state one important lesson they have learned from the session. It is important that there is time left for players to de-role.

# Variants of role play

## Video role play

Here the pair are videoed role playing a scenario and the positive critique and feedback subsequently occur on a one-to-one basis with the facilitator.

## Role play in pairs or trios

This allows all the members of a group to take part either as a pair of role players or as two role players and an observer. Once the steps for role play in a small group have been followed, they go to different rooms, or to different parts of a large room, and quietly practise the role play together, with no audience other than the observer. The facilitator's role is to circulate and be available in case people become stuck with their role play.

We find this a very good technique to use during a study day when people have already practised other techniques in the teaching communication skills ladder but want a chance to actually do some communicating themselves without an audience. It is less threatening than the small group form of role play.

## What to watch out for

⚠ People often have negative past experience of role play.

⚠ The second facilitator looks out for signs of stress in any of the learners and can call time out.

⚠ It is important for the facilitator not to let the role play go on too long as points can be missed and participants begin to struggle.

⚠ Role play should not be more difficult than real life.

⚠ The facilitator needs to use his or her skill to make sure everyone contributes.

⚠ Role play can be tiring for participants.

⚠ The session may need lifting at the end. A lighthearted game or icebreaker can help.

⚠ Offer an opportunity to talk to a facilitator alone later.

⚠ Never forget to de-role.

# Sculpting

Sculpting is a form of dynamic non-verbal role play in which participants are arranged in positions, which symbolise feelings, conflicts and power relationships. It is a technique which originated as a form of family therapy.[11] In this setting the members of a family are represented in positions symbolising the relationships between them. A family member creates a sculpture by arranging the other members in a way which physically represents their interpersonal relationships. Aspects of relationships such as loving, conflict, loss, power and status can thus be depicted spatially in terms of distance or closeness. The positions can be altered in the light of different participants' perceptions.

This is a technique which can be used:

• to improve communication skills

• to explore family relationships

• to enhance team working.

## How to do it

The technique involves a small group of participants, ideally no more than 12, and two facilitators. It is important that the facilitators are comfortable with experiential learning methods and, particularly, role play. One facilitator takes a lead in conducting the sculpt, the other has the task of detecting any signs of distress amongst the participants and calling a pause to the activity, if appropriate, to protect group members.

⇒ Introductions.

⇒ Icebreaker.

⇒ The aims of the session are clearly listed on a flip chart.

⇒ A facilitator describes the technique of sculpting.

⇒ Participants are asked if they have any previous experience of either sculpting or role play. They have an opportunity to describe, first, positive and then any negative past experiences.

⇒ The facilitator negotiates groundrules for the session.

⇒ The facilitator describes a clinical situation, which may have come from the participants or been brought to the group by the facilitator.

⇒ Roles are assigned to the participants.

⇒ The facilitator checks that this scenario is appropriate to explore for all members of the group.

⇒ Participants get into position.

⇒ Each participant reflects on how this feels.

⇒ Verbal feedback to group.

⇒ Dynamic repositioning.

⇒ Further reflection.

⇒ Verbal feedback.

⇒ Group conclusion.

⇒ De-role.

⇒ Evaluation.

## What to watch out for

The method and purpose need to be carefully explained to participants who might otherwise think it bizarre. Sculpting is a powerful way of exploring feelings and emotions that participants may not express in a verbal communications exercise.

It may be that the story inadvertently triggers some personal experience for a group member. If this is the case a substitute clinical situation should be set up.

It is vital that the participants and facilitators feel safe and trust each other. Sculpting should only be carried out within a group whose members are already familiar with each other – for example, GP Registrars on a vocational training scheme, a primary care team, or attendees on a one or two day course on communication skills. This technique should not be used to fill in an hour's teaching slot on communication skills.

## Sculpting: an example

*Topic*: **Teamwork in the care of a dying patient**

*Aim*: To gain insights into the advantages and challenges of multidisciplinary teamwork.

John is a 55-year old teacher with advanced cancer of the prostate with bone and liver metastases. He has had surgery, radiotherapy and hormone treatment and is aware that there are no further treatment options for the cancer. He lives at home with his wife Jill, aged 50, who retired from community nursing because of severe asthma. They have one son, Derek (28), who lives close by. John is deteriorating day by day; he spends much of the time in bed. He is taking morphine for his back pain but still has disturbed nights. He has constipation and finds using the commode increasingly difficult. He has expressed the wish that he would like to remain at home to die.

**TEACHING PLAN**

✓ The facilitator checks that this scenario is appropriate for all members of the group.

✓ The group 'brainstorm' the people they feel would be available to support John and his family. The facilitator lists these on a flip chart. Responses might include:

- community nurse
- general practitioner
- Macmillan nurse
- Marie Curie nurse
- home care assistant
- neighbour
- palliative medicine consultant
- priest
- social worker.

✓ One member of the group volunteers to be John. Other members are allocated one of the roles listed. Participants are given a minute to imagine their roles.

✓ John then sits (or lies on a couch) and places each person around the room in a position which he feels best meets his needs.

✓ The facilitator checks that John is happy with the arrangement and then asks each of the participants in role to say how they feel about the position that John has placed them in. Typical comments might be:

*See overleaf*

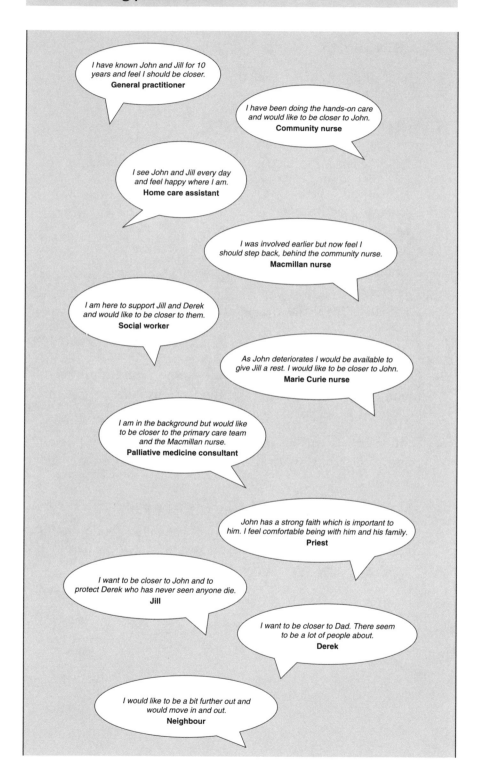

✓ After each person has spoken they are allowed to move to a position which they feel more accurately symbolises their role in the care of the patient and family.

✓ The participants again have a chance to say whether they now feel more comfortable and the family then responds to the changes.

✓ At the end of the sculpt the facilitator de-roles the participants. A group discussion identifies learning points which can be summarised on the flip chart by the facilitator.

In this sculpt the patient said he felt well supported but also a bit crowded by the professionals. The professionals appreciated the risk of denying John his privacy. The professionals whom the patient selects as key workers may not coincide with the professional view.

The professionals also had a chance to see where they could get support and advice and how important it is to co-ordinate visits so that not too many people are in the house at the same time. The differing roles of the community nurse, Macmillan nurse and the Marie Curie nurse can also be explored in the context of the positions they have adopted.

# Chapter 8

# Evaluation

Evaluation measures the effectiveness of different parts of the educational process, for example, the performance of the teacher. It is not the same as assessment, which measures the attainments and achievements of learners in terms of their knowledge, skills and attitudes.

Evaluation of an education programme involves much more than filling in a short questionnaire. In evaluating an education programme we need to answer five questions.

1  Why is the evaluation required?
2  Who should do the evaluation?
3  What aspects of the programme should be evaluated?
4  What kind of measurement will be used?
5  When will it be done?

# Why is the evaluation required?

- To justify expenditure.
- To allow feedback to the trainers.
- To enable improvements to be made to the programme.
- Evaluation is an essential part of the learning cycle.
- To measure whether learning objectives have been met.

# Who should do the evaluation?

Evaluation is a joint process between the teacher and the learner. The learner should reflect on issues such as:

- how well did I prepare for the teaching session?
- how much did I contribute to the session?
- had I clearly thought about my own learning needs?
- what measures have I incorporated to achieve these learning needs?
- how will the educational experience alter my practice in the future?

The teacher should reflect on issues such as:

- did I plan and prepare the teaching adequately?
- did I clearly state the aims and learning outcomes for the session?
- did I assess the needs of the learners?
- was the time planning appropriate?
- did everyone get an opportunity to contribute?
- did everyone get a chance to give verbal feedback?
- how do I know if my teaching has been successful?

If there are clearly stated learning objectives and aims for each teaching session, then it is easier to measure whether these objectives have been achieved. It is more difficult to assess whether teaching has influenced attitudes, beliefs and values and thus affected clinical practice.

# What aspects of the programme should be evaluated?

All aspects of the education process can be evaluated, for example:

- the performance of the teacher
- the teacher's presentation skills
- the level of interest maintained in the topic
- the clinical relevance of the topic
- the environment of the education
- the quality of the AV equipment
- participants' ability to rest
- participants' ability to interact with other participants.

# What kind of measurement will be used?

A verbal evaluation can be undertaken by the participants at the course as a closing exercise. Each person might be asked to identify one thing that they have taken from the course which will alter their practice in the future.

A written evaluation gives the learner time to reflect and write a freehand evaluation of aspects of the course using the principles of positive critique, i.e. identifying things that were good before commenting on things which could be improved. A value or attitudinal rating scale may be used. This can be a visual analogue scale where learners mark their degree of agreement or disagreement with a stem sentence.

# When will it be done?

Depending on the subject material, it is probably most practical to evaluate a session immediately. However, this does not allow for reflection. It may be more useful to carry out some form of distant evaluation such as a questionnaire completed 2 or 3 months after the session, or an interview with participants 2 or 3 months after the session.

# What to do with the evaluation

The teachers involved need to receive the evaluation and have a chance to meet together to discuss the information.

Initially we discuss what has gone well. In addition to the feedback from the learners, if team teaching is used there is always positive feedback from your co-teacher. It can be helpful to have a colleague just listing the competencies that you have displayed during the teaching. Another alternative which we are contemplating, but have not used yet, would be to video the teacher. The video could then be used to demonstrate competencies.

In the spirit of positive critique it is only once we have exhausted all the positive aspects of the teaching that we move to looking at aspects which could have been improved. The teacher first has an opportunity to say what he/she thinks could have been improved. After discussion the co-teacher then gives his/her suggestions for improvement.

Whilst it is true that you will never please everybody, it is important to reflect on the negative as well as the positive.

## An evaluation form from a PEGG Study Day

Evaluation of 'What is Palliative Care?' Study Day

Held on 17 June 1999 at The Sue Ryder Palliative Care Home, Cheltenham

Were you able to hear all the speakers?    Yes ☐    No ☐

If no, please note the specific speakers you had difficulty hearing.

| *Please score the sessions (1–5)* | | Poor | | | | Excellent |
|---|---|---|---|---|---|---|
| Definition of palliative care | *Presentation* | 1 | 2 | 3 | 4 | 5 |
| | *Content* | 1 | 2 | 3 | 4 | 5 |
| | *Interest* | 1 | 2 | 3 | 4 | 5 |
| Cancer journey | *Presentation* | 1 | 2 | 3 | 4 | 5 |
| | *Content* | 1 | 2 | 3 | 4 | 5 |
| | *Interest* | 1 | 2 | 3 | 4 | 5 |
| Needs of patients, families and staff | *Presentation* | 1 | 2 | 3 | 4 | 5 |
| | *Content* | 1 | 2 | 3 | 4 | 5 |
| | *Interest* | 1 | 2 | 3 | 4 | 5 |
| Teamwork – who does what | *Presentation* | 1 | 2 | 3 | 4 | 5 |
| | *Content* | 1 | 2 | 3 | 4 | 5 |
| | *Interest* | 1 | 2 | 3 | 4 | 5 |
| I don't know what to say (Communication issues) | *Presentation* | 1 | 2 | 3 | 4 | 5 |
| | *Content* | 1 | 2 | 3 | 4 | 5 |
| | *Interest* | 1 | 2 | 3 | 4 | 5 |
| So what now? (Bereavement issues) | *Presentation* | 1 | 2 | 3 | 4 | 5 |
| | *Content* | 1 | 2 | 3 | 4 | 5 |
| | *Interest* | 1 | 2 | 3 | 4 | 5 |

We hope you have enjoyed the workshops. Please help us by giving any further comments.

# Chapter 9

# Training the trainers

An integral part of the PEGG programme is a two-day course to teach teachers how to improve their own teaching skills. The multidisciplinary team teaching approach adopted by PEGG means that in every teaching situation, less experienced teachers have the opportunity to work alongside experienced colleagues. When they have gained in confidence they in turn lead a session alongside a less experienced teacher alongside.

# Training the trainers: Day 1

9:00–9:30    REGISTRATION AND COFFEE

This gives the 12 participants a chance to meet each other and to meet our PEGG administrator. Each participant has received a programme for the day and has made a commitment to attend both training days. The course is held in a hotel or conference centre to allow clinicians to get out of their working environment and relax. Mobile phones are prohibited during the teaching sessions.

9:30–10:15    INTRODUCTION

Usually a simple icebreaker. The 12 participants meet the three (or four) facilitators. It is important that there are at least three facilitators for this course and we generally prefer four. During the introduction groundrules are set.

*Aims of the day*

- To identify what is a good teaching experience.
- To identify and share what we find difficult in teaching.
- To improve our teaching skills.

- To have a chance to practise teaching.
- To gain confidence in our ability to teach.
- To have fun!

We explain to the participants that there will be times during the course when they will be asked to act as a group of doctors/nurses/ social workers attending a communication skills course. Various teaching sessions will be held and they are to participate as if they were attending to improve their own communication skills. At the end of a teaching session, which might only be partly completed, they will step out of this role and become themselves, i.e. healthcare professionals learning how to teach.

The facilitator who was conducting the demonstration teaching session then hands over to an identified educational facilitator whose role is to lead a discussion on the teaching techniques, competencies and formats that were used. This discussion is, as always, informed by positive critique.

We find it helpful to have two flip charts for the course with two different coloured pens. One chart is used during the demonstration teaching and the other is reserved for summarising the educational aspects of the session.

Having checked that all the participants are happy with this split role, we proceed with the agenda.

Participants go into pairs or trios to describe a good learning experience. Often they will remember a teacher from their school days. Various factors are noted on the flip chart.

Next we explore the reasons why clinicians find teaching difficult. This discussion, which may be conducted in pairs or trios, often uncovers previous bad learning experiences.

We summarise this part of the day by saying we will strive to enhance what is good and give people the confidence to get over any blocks to teaching. The simple exercise of sharing difficulties is often empowering. We all have difficulties and even the teachers who appear most competent and confident are often trembling jellies inside!

10:15–11:00  ADULT LEARNING MODELS:
HOW DO WE LEARN?

It is a great advantage to have the contribution of a professional educator in the team. A little educational theory helps teachers to assess the learners' needs and gives them confidence. This is an interactive session with graphic video illustrations of learning by humiliation (or more accurately, not learning by humiliation), discussions of adult learning and the use of learning style questionnaires.

11:00–11:30  COFFEE

Allow plenty of time for coffee and for those who need to use their mobile phones.

11:30–12:30  COMMUNICATION SKILLS: THE LADDER

After a brief description of our approach to teaching communication skills, two facilitators start a teaching session using an interactive video. After 30 minutes the educational facilitator interrupts the session at an appropriate point. He/she tells the group that they are now teachers. The facilitators comment on what went well. The learner–teachers then add their positive contributions before looking at ways of improving the session.

12:30–1:30  LUNCH

Find a location where the food is good! Participants eat and chat together. The facilitators use the time for a shorter lunch, reflection, fine-tune planning and sharing any concerns.

| | |
|---|---|
| 2:00–2:20 | **THE USE OF ROLE PLAY** |

The group are given a chance to talk about their experiences of role play. Sadly, these are more commonly negative rather than positive. The theory and principles are discussed.

| | |
|---|---|
| 2:20–3:00 | **GOLDFISH BOWL** |

A facilitator puts two other facilitators into role and carries out a goldfish bowl demonstration session. The session is stopped by the (fourth) educational facilitator and the group then discuss the technique.

| | |
|---|---|
| 3:00–3:15 | **TEA** |

| | |
|---|---|
| 3:15–4:10 | **ROLE PLAY** |

One of the facilitators sets the scene for a short role play which can be done in pairs, not in front of an audience. Here the participants role play in pairs for about 10 minutes. Three facilitators are available to help. Discussion about using role play in this unthreatening atmosphere is followed by suggestions for improvements.

| | |
|---|---|
| 4:10–4:30 | **EVALUATION & THOUGHTS ON THE PROGRAMME FOR DAY 2** |

A written and verbal evaluation of the day are followed by a brief discussion on the content of the programme for Day 2. Participants are encouraged to contact the facilitators if they think of other issues that they would like to cover. Sometimes these are too involved to incorporate into the programme. For instance, one group wanted to have a session on videoing consultations as a teaching technique. We felt that we would need a whole day to cover this important topic adequately.

The day ends with a humorous video clip.

# Training the trainers: Day 2

9:00–9:30     REGISTRATION AND COFFEE

Day 2 is usually held 2 months after Day 1 to give participants a chance to teach and reflect on whether the course has helped them. This morning break allows the group to reform and to share some of their experiences.

9:30–9:45     GROUNDRULES AND CHECKING THE AGENDA

The participants discuss the plan for the day and raise any concerns.

9:45–10:45     TEACHING TECHNIQUES

There is an opportunity to revisit the teaching techniques covered in Day 1, to share what has gone well, and to discuss a few techniques, e.g. icebreakers, illustrations or video clips that people have found to be successful.

10:45–11:15     COFFEE

11:15–12:30     SCULPTING

This form of role play was described in Chapter 7. It is a new technique which stimulates a great deal of interest.

Some groups have had so much teaching since the Day 1 course that they have needed extra time in the morning to share their teaching experiences with the group.

12:30–1:30     LUNCH

1:30–3:00   PLANNING A TEACHING SESSION

The participants split into three groups of four people and plan one of the following:

- a two-hour session for junior hospital doctors on breaking bad news
- a study day on handling uncertainty in palliative care
- an afternoon teaching session for GPs and community nurses on talking to patients with advanced cancer.

The groups have 45 minutes to plan the session and 10 minutes to feed back to the whole group. Each group gets positive feedback on their plan from their colleagues.

3:00–3:15   TEA

3:15–4:00   EVALUATION: ARE WE EFFECTIVE TEACHERS?

A brief discussion of the principles of evaluation, followed by a review of techniques for evaluation.

4:00–4:30   CONCLUSION

A chance to reflect on the two days and to deal with unresolved issues. For example, one group wanted to deal with problem participants. The group discussed tactics for managing silent, hostile or bored participants in small group teaching.

# Chapter 10

# Lesson plans

To draw together parts of the practical toolbox, we include some lesson plans from the PEGG programme to illustrate how we select teaching techniques.

# Lesson plan: What is palliative care?

Plan for the day for 20 multiprofessional non-clinical staff.

| | |
|---|---|
| 09:00–09:30 | REGISTRATION |
| 09:30–09:45 | INTRODUCTIONS/ICEBREAKER |

09:30–09:45 INTRODUCTIONS/ICEBREAKER
Say who you are, where you work and a nice thing that happened to you this morning.

09:45–11:00 SET GROUNDRULES

*What are the problems?*
- OHP 1: A definition of palliative care
- OHP 2: The cancer journey

*Icebreaker 2*

What situations do you find difficult in dealing with cancer patients or their relatives?

The participants separate into trios or pairs. Their tasks are to identify:
- why it is difficult
- the feelings this difficulty arouses in them
- the feelings shown by the patient or relative.

This is a 20-minute exercise. Feedback to a flip chart.

*Case scenario*

An OHP is used to display a genogram. A man has prostate cancer. He is aged 60, and married to Betty. They have two sons, Jim and Peter. Peter is married with two sons. What are the patient's and family's needs?

Split into trios to identify physical, social, psychological and spiritual needs.

11:00        COFFEE

11:30–12:45  MEETING THE NEEDS – TEAMWORK
             *Brainstorm*
             What are the positive aspects about working in a team? What are the difficulties? These are drawn up on the flip chart.

             *Short presentation: what is a team?*
             OHPs are used to depict what a team is, the various people involved in the team, overlapping roles, who makes up the team in palliative care, who the local members of the palliative care team are.

             *Introduction to local specialist services*

12:45        LUNCH

1:30–3:00    COMMUNICATION ISSUES
             The topic for this session may be taken from one of the difficult situations described in the morning. During the lunch break the facilitators get together and arrange a goldfish bowl for the afternoon session.

             *Goldfish bowl*
             Betty, Fred's wife, rang the receptionist at the hospital as Fred's outpatient appointment had been postponed for two weeks. The reason for cancellation is that the consultant is away from the hospital giving a teaching session so will be unavailable for the whole day. One person is a

facilitator, another plays the receptionist, Sharon, and another plays Betty, the patient's wife. A second situation was discussed: relatives arriving on the ward before a death certificate was ready. Again this was enacted as a goldfish bowl situation.

## TEA

## EVALUATION AND CLOSING EXERCISE

Each member of the group says one thing that they have learned from the day and how this will alter their practice in the future. They then complete a formal evaluation form.

As a closing exercise, everyone should say one nice thing that they are looking forward to doing in the evening.

# Lesson plan: Pain control

Plan for the day for 20 qualified staff from hospital and the community.

Facilitated by:

- Specialist Nurse from the Palliative Care Team
- Consultant in Palliative Care
- Community Macmillan Nurse
- Psychologist.

Aims of the day:

- to gain a clear understanding of the different physiology and different types of cancer pain
- to understand the different methods of pain assessment
- to gain understanding and knowledge in pain management using the WHO analgesic ladder
- to devise a stepwise approach to the management of bone and neuropathic pain
- to gain a practical knowledge of syringe drivers and TENS machines
- to understand the concept of total pain.

9:00–9:15    REGISTRATION AND COFFEE

9:15–9:30    INTRODUCTION OF FACILITATORS AND
             SIMPLE ICEBREAKER

- What is your name?
- Where do you work?
- Say one thing which makes you unique in
  this group.

A simple questionnaire on the WHO ladder and analgesics is
handed out to be completed by all the participants.

9:30–10:15   DIFFERENT TYPES OF CANCER PAIN

             A group discussion on the different types of
             cancer pain, and presentation using OHPs and
             flip chart. The concept of pain and the
             analgesic ladder.

10:15–10:45  PAIN ASSESSMENTS

             Methods described on OHPs as a straight
             presentation from the specialist nurse.

10:45–11:15  COFFEE

11:15–12:45  PAIN MANAGEMENT

             Participants split into three small groups, each
             to discuss one of the following:

- a case of bone pain
- a case of neuropathic pain
- a case of visceral pain.

             20 minutes to discuss the case management
             and then 10 minutes to present the findings.

12:45–1:30   LUNCH

| | |
|---|---|
| 1:30–2:10 | **SYRINGE DRIVERS AND TENS**<br>Participants divide into five small groups and rotate between syringe drivers and TENS machines for a practical session. |
| 2:10–3:00 | **PSYCHOLOGY OF PAIN**<br>A Powerpoint presentation with interactive elements. |
| 3:00–3:15 | **TEA** |
| 3:15–3:45 | **HOT TOPICS IN PALLIATIVE CARE**<br>Opioid switching: a group discussion with overheads on one or two new drugs. |
| 3:45–4:00 | **EVALUATION AND CLOSE**<br>Second completion of the pain questionnaire; evaluation questionnaire; participants share something they have learned and something they look forward to doing at the weekend. |

# Lesson plan: Breaking bad news

Plan for the day for 20 qualified staff from hospital and the community.

Facilitated by:

- Specialist Nurse from the Palliative Care Team
- Consultant in Palliative Care
- Hospital Chaplain
- Macmillan Social Worker
- Psychologist.

Aims of the day:

- to improve our communication skills
- to identify difficult issues in talking to patients and relatives
- to improve our confidence by practising our communication skills.

09:00–09:15   REGISTRATION AND COFFEE

09:15–09:30   INTRODUCTION AND ICEBREAKER

A short video clip from the film *One Hundred and One Dalmatians* illustrating difficulties in communication.

Set each participant to talk to the person sitting next to them and ask them to introduce their neighbour to the rest of the group.

09:30–10:45   ISSUES SURROUNDING BREAKING BAD NEWS

Participants split into trios and discuss difficult situations they have faced, why it was difficult and how the situations affected them and the recipients of the bad news.

This is fed back and the difficult issues are then discussed.

10:45–11:00 COFFEE

11:00–12:45 HOW CAN WE IMPROVE BREAKING BAD NEWS?

Interactive video of a consultant breaking bad news to a patient with cervical cancer, reiterating the need for positive critique.

12:45–2:00 LUNCH

2:00–3:00 PRACTISING OUR COMMUNICATION SKILLS

Goldfish bowl role play on breaking bad news of a diagnosis of inoperable pancreatic cancer to a young man.

3:00–3:15 TEA

3:15–4:15 WHAT WOULD MAKE YOU CHANGE PRACTICE?

A group discussion on the process of breaking bad news, supplemented by illustrations from videos and short group exercises such as the eye contact game.

4:15 EVALUATION AND CLOSE

# Chapter 11

# Conclusions

The PEGG education programme aims to inspire healthcare professionals to think, to reflect and to improve their professional judgements. Working in palliative care involves working with colleagues from different disciplines in clinical situations filled with uncertainty. Specialists in palliative care have a responsibility to enable their colleagues to deliver a high standard of care to patients with cancer.

Education is a process of facilitation whereby the teacher recognises the potential within the learner and provides that vital spark which ignites the desire to learn. The learner becomes responsible for their own education and, in learning, seeks to understand. It is this understanding which is the ultimate value in education.

Healthcare professionals need space, time and a supportive atmosphere in which to learn to understand. PEGG programmes attempt to provide this in several ways:

- by limiting the numbers
- by employing groundrules
- by applying positive critique
- and by encouraging clinicians to see every clinical contact as an opportunity to gain understanding.

If learning is to take place, we need to create an environment where even experienced professionals can express their doubts and feelings of vulnerability without feeling inadequate.

Clinicians are firmly anchored in practice. Teaching must acknowledge this and has to be relevant. The teacher needs to ascertain the learner's needs and then negotiate clear learning objectives. This emphasis on relevance of teaching material is reflected in modern 'problem-oriented' curricula in medical schools.

In a learning environment facilitated by enthusiastic, yet sensitive, teachers and a philosophy of positive critique, learners may flourish. They become willing to examine their own knowledge, attitudes and experience. They become reflective practitioners.

The questions they ask of themselves become more sophisticated, moving from 'What do I do now?' to 'What ought I to do now?'

Working with uncertainty requires professionals to assess a situation, adopt a flexible approach, listen to others and make professional judgements when there is no right answer. This combination of clinical competence and common sense has been called practical wisdom or professional artistry.

How can we continue to foster this climate of learning? We can start by extending our groundrules and philosophy of positive critique into our working practice. We need to value our colleagues, from whichever discipline, and ensure that they feel part of the same learning community. We need to allow time for reflection on our practice and to see appraisal as a mechanism by which we can grow in understanding. There needs to be recognition that 'education, education, education' is not simply a political slogan but the way in which the care of patients is going to improve. Education needs resources and recognition that it is part of the everyday work of the many who are concerned with the patient.

The word doctor is derived from the latin 'docere', which means 'to teach'. We hope that this practical guide encourages our colleagues to share their skills and uncertainties, in other words . . . to teach.

# References

1 World Health Organization (1990) *Cancer Pain Relief and Palliative Care.* WHO Technical Report Series 804. WHO, Geneva.

2 Dunlop RJ and Hockley JM (1998) *Hospital-based Palliative Care Teams.* Oxford University Press, Oxford.

3 Keogh K, Jeffrey D and Flanagan S (1999) The Palliative Care Education Group for Gloucestershire (PEGG): an integrated model of multidisciplinary education in palliative care. *European Journal of Cancer Care.* 8: 44–7.

4 Pietroni R (1992) New strategies for higher professional education. *British Journal of General Practice.* 42: 294–6.

5 Knowles MS (1980) *The Modern Practice of Adult Education: from pedagogy to andragogy* (2e). Cambridge Books, New York.

6 Knowles MS (1984) *Andragogy in Action: applying modern principles of adult learning.* Jossey-Bass, San Francisco.

7 Jeffrey D (1994) Education in palliative care: a qualitative evaluation of the present state and the needs of general practitioners and community nurses. *European Journal of Cancer Care.* 3: 67–74.

8 Barclay S, Todd C, Grande G and Lipscombe J (1997) How common is medical training in palliative care? A postal survey of general practitioners. *British Journal of General Practice.* 47: 800–5.

9 Macleod RD and Nash A (1991) Teaching palliative care in general practice: a survey of educational needs and preferences. *Journal of Palliative Care.* 7: 9–12.

10 Greenhalgh T (1997) How to read a paper: the basics of evidence-based medicine. *British Medical Journal.* 315: 243–6.

11 Kantor D and Duhl BS (1973) Learning, space and action in family therapy: a primer of sculpture. In: D Bloch (ed.) *Techniques of Family Psychotherapy: a primer.* Grine & Stratton, New York.

# Index

active process, learning as 6, 9–10
aims
  PEGG 93–5
  teaching 9
  of this book 2–3
assumptions, learning 6–7
atmosphere groundrule 23
audio-visual (AV) equipment 17–19

bad news, breaking
  lesson plan 90–1
  mannequin, teaching technique 28
ball catching, teaching technique 24
bedside teaching *see* clinical bedside
  teaching
book/picture/music, teaching technique
  26

cards, teaching technique 24–5
case-control studies, critiquing a paper
  30
case reports, critiquing a paper 30
chairpersons
  debates 35
  lectures 34
changing seats, teaching technique 24
checklist, study day 14–15
clinical bedside teaching
  example 41–2
  how to do it 40
  teaching format 16
  teaching plan 41–2
  teaching technique 39–42
  what to watch out for 40
clinical supervision
  defined 42
  *see also* supervision
cliques 24
cohort studies, critiquing a paper 30

communication
  barriers 21
  eye contact 27–8, 45
  non-verbal 28
  *see also* sculpting
communication skills ladder, teaching
  technique 49–57
computer projection, AV equipment
  18–19
conclusions 93–8
conference presentations, AV equipment
  18
confidentiality groundrule 23
  clinical bedside teaching 40
  mentoring 43
creative activities, teaching technique
  25–6
critique groundrule 23
critiquing a paper
  journal clubs 31
  presentation type 29, 30–1
cross-sectional surveys, critiquing a paper
  30

debates
  points to remember 36
  presentation type 29, 35–6
difficult audiences, lectures 33

education process 94
environment, teaching and learning 3,
  6–7, 9, 94–5
equipment, audio-visual 17–19
evaluation 69–74
  aspects for evaluation 71
  feedback 72–3
  form 73
  learners and 7
  measurement types 72

participants 70–1
reason for 70
timing of 72
evidence hierarchies 30
eye contact, and communication 27–8,
45

facilitating skills
example 45–6
how to do it 45
single facilitation cf. double facilitation
44
in small group teaching 44–8
what to watch out for 47–8
formats, teaching 16

goldfish bowl technique
communication skills 50, 53–7
example 55
how to do it 54–5
teaching plan 56
groundrules, teaching techniques 22–3
group teaching *see* small group teaching

hands across the world, teaching
technique 25
honesty groundrule 23

icebreakers, teaching technique 23–4
illustration, teaching technique 26–7
informal talks, value of 20
interactive video *see* video, interactive
involving learners 7

journal clubs
running 31
teaching format 16

learners
evaluation and 70–1
'good' 8
involving 7
needs, identifying 15
planning benefits 13
learning
as an active process 6, 9–10
assumptions 6–7
environment 3, 6–7, 9, 94–5

ethos 7
passive 7
principles 5–8
specific needs 6
lectures
AV equipment 18
chairpersons 34
difficult audiences 33
how to lecture 32
points to remember 33
presentation type 29, 32–5
teaching format 16
lesson plans 83–98
breaking bad news 90–1
pain control 87–9
palliative care described 84–6

mentoring
groundrules 43
how to do it 43–4
learner's responsibilities 43
role of mentor 42–3
teaching technique 42–4
meta-analyses, critiquing a paper 30
methodology, critiquing a paper 30–1
multidisciplinary palliative care,
defined 1

needs, identifying learners' 15
newspaper articles, teaching technique
25–6
non-verbal communication 28
*see also* sculpting

OHPs *see* overhead projectors
one-to-one teaching, teaching technique
37–48
organising 11–20
overhead projectors (OHPs) 17–19, 26–7

Palliative Care Education Group of
Gloucestershire (PEGG) 2–3
aims 93–5
evaluation form 73
philosophy 9–10
training the trainers 76–81

palliative care, multidisciplinary,
     defined 1
PEGG *see* Palliative Care Education
     Group of Gloucestershire
perfect palliator, teaching technique 25
physical activities, teaching technique
     24–5
planning 11–20
  AV equipment 17–19
  checklist, study day 14–15
  decisions 15–17
  evaluation 20
  last minute fine-tuning 20
  learners' benefits 13
  meeting agenda 14
  objectives 12
  priorities 13
  a study day 13–15
  time spent 12
practical exercises, teaching technique
     27–8
presentations 29–36
  example 34–5
  types 29
primary research 30
principles, learning 5–8

qualities, teachers 8–9

randomised controlled trials, critiquing a
     paper 30
references 97–8
research, primary/secondary 30
respect for others groundrule 23
role play
  communication skills 50, 60–2
  how to do it 60–1
  pairs or trios 61
  variants 61–2
  what to watch out for 62
  *see also* sculpting

sculpting
  communication skills 50, 62–7
  example 64–7
  how to do it 63

teaching plan 65–7
  what to watch out for 64
secondary research 30
seminar, teaching format 16
slides, AV equipment 18–19, 26–7
small group teaching
  AV equipment 18
  facilitating skills in 44–8
  teaching format 16
  teaching technique 37–48
supervision
  teaching format 16
  teaching technique 42–4
systematic reviews, critiquing a paper 30

teachers
  evaluation and 70–1
  as facilitators 9
  'good' 8–9
  qualities 8–9
  training 75–81
teaching
  aim 9
  approach 5–10
  didactic cf. experiental 7
  environment 3, 6–7, 9, 94–5
  formats 16
  inhibitions to 1–2
teaching material, relevance 6
teaching techniques
  choice of 15–16
  communication skills ladder 49–57
  creative activities 25–6
  icebreakers 23–4, 45
  illustration 26–7
  introductions 21–8
  one-to-one teaching 37–48
  physical activities 24–5
  practical exercises 27–8
  presentations 29–36
  role play 50, 60–2
  sculpting 50, 62–7
  small group teaching 37–48
teamworking 9, 62
techniques, teaching 15–16
time out groundrule 23
training, training the trainers 75–81
true or false, teaching technique 26

tutorials
  example 39
  teaching format 16
tutoring
  how to do it 38
  teaching technique 38
  what to watch out for 38

uncertainty envelope, teaching technique
  28

venue, teaching 17
video, AV equipment 18–19, 26–7
video, interactive
  communication skills 50–3
  example 52–3
  facilitator's checklist 52
  how to do it 51–2
video, role play 61

workshop, teaching format 16